Big Momma's Hands

RayeQueen

Dedication

Our ancestors provided us a blueprint for optimal health and wellness. This information was designed to be handed down from generation to generation to ensure our continued vitality. Given honor to the Most High, the ancestors, my grandmother, and my mother, my work exists because of you

Big Momma's Hands

RayeQueen

First published in United States in 2018 by
RayeQueen

Table of Contents

Introduction

This book is written for the everyday person looking for time proven natural, herbal, nutritional, vitamin, juice, and alternative remedies to treat, manage, and reverse many of the health ailments and diseases that has affected many generations at such alarming rates. Although the modern world would have you believe that these remedies are 'alternative' they are actually remedies that our ancestors used to sustain our lineages for thousands of years. Use it!

This is a simple and straightforward book intended for the everyday person to use. Carry it with you at the health food store as you look for natural remedies. Incorporate as many food and vitamin recommendations your heart desires but only choose 1 herbal remedy at a time. Allow 30 days before switching to another.

Dosage

When you purchase vitamins, herbs or minerals basic dosage rules will be included on the package but it will also say 'or as directed by your healthcare practitioner'. I am your healthcare practitioner! A good rule to follow is if you are taking vitamins or herbs as a preventive measure, follow the dosage on the bottle. If you are treating a current condition, increase the dosage by half. If you are taking prescription medicine, please check with your healthcare practitioner for interactions.

ABSCESS

Nutritional Therapy

- Fresh filtered water
- Avoid refined sugars and alcohol for two weeks
- Avoid cow's milk
- Avoid processed foods

Vitamin/Mineral Therapy

- Vitamin A (50,000 IU for two weeks)
- Beta Carotene (100,000 IU for two weeks)
- Zinc (60 mg daily for two weeks)
- Vitamin C (2,000 mg daily)
- Lactobacillus acidophilus (several times daily)

Herbal Therapy

- Garlic
- Burdock root
- Cayenne
- Red clover

Homeopathy

- Belladonna
- Hepar sulph
- Silicea

Topical Treatment

- Calendula ointment
- Apply vitamin A capsule (10,000 IU)
- Apply liquid chlorophyll

<u>ACNE</u>

Nutritional Therapy
- Eat plenty of vegetables
- Eat whole fruits
- Reduce animal fats
- Minimize caffeine, sugars, and alcohol
- Increase fiber
- Fast one day a week

Vitamin Therapy
- Vitamin A (10,000 IU daily for two weeks)
- Beta Carotene (50,000 IU for one month)
- B Complex Vitamins
- Vitamin C (1,000 mg three times daily)
- Vitamin E (800 IU daily)

Herbal Therapy
- Sarsaparilla
- Burdock
- Calendula
- Chamomile

Homeopathy
- Pulsatilla
- Sulfur

Juice Therapy
- Carrot, beet and celery
- Carrot, cucumber, lettuce, spinach

ADDICTIONS

Food Therapy

- Eat protein with every meal

Vitamin/Mineral Therapy

- Zinc
- Vitamin C
- Chromium
- Choline
- Folic Acid

Herbal Therapy

- Milk Thistle
- Dandelion
- Oat Straw

Homeopathy

- Berberis
- Nux vomica
- Sulphur
- Lachesis

ANXIETY

Nutritional Therapy
- Avoid excessive consumption of refined sugars
- Avoid cow's milk
- Eat broth
- Eat nuts and seeds

Vitamin/Mineral Therapy
- Calcium
- Magnesium
- Vitamin B complex

Herbal Therapy
- Gaba
- Panax ginseng
- Valerian
- Kava kava
- St. John's Wort

Homeopathy
- Aconite
- Actaea rac.
- Sulfur

<u>ATHLETE'S FOOT</u>

Nutritional Therapy
- Raw foods
- Less dairy products
- Avoid foods with yeast
- Avoid sugars

Vitamin/Mineral Therapy
- Vitamin B Complex
- Vitamin C (2,000 mg. daily)
- Vitamin E
- Vitamin A

Herbal Therapy
- Garlic Capsules

Homeopathy
- Calendula
- Chamomilla
- Belladonna

Juice Therapy
- Add garlic to vegetable juice

Topical Therapy
- Apply tea tree oil
- Apply citrus seed extract
- Apply apple cider vinegar

AIDS

Nutritional Therapy

- Eat organic fruits and vegetables with minimal cooking
- Avoid processed food
- Reduce or eliminate refined carbohydrates
- Reduce or eliminate unhealthy fats and oils. Use olive oil or Coconut oil. (consume coconut oil daily).
- Eat smaller portions of food more frequently
- Eliminate chocolate, caffeine, and alcohol

Vitamin/Mineral Therapy

- Vitamin A
- B Complex
- Vitamin C
- Vitamin E
- Potassium
- Magnesium
- Manganese
- Omega 3's and omega 6's
- Selenium

Herbal Therapy

- Astragalus
- Echinacea
- Licorice
- Goldenseal

Other

- Oxygen therapy
- Periods of increased body temperatures above 98.6°

ALZHEIMER'S DISEASE

Nutritional Therapy
- Eat adequate amounts of protein
- Do not eat foods with artificial coloring
- Do not cook with aluminum

Vitamin/Mineral Therapy
- Coenzyme Q10
- Vitamin B6
- Vitamin C
- Evening Primrose
- Zinc
- Selenium

Herbal Therapy
- Ginkgo Biloba

Other
- Exercise
- Stop Smoking

<u>ARTHRITIS</u>

Nutritional Therapy
- Eat whole foods
- Avoid processed foods

Vitamins/Minerals Therapy
- Vitamin C
- Vitamin A
- Vitamin B1
- Vitamin B6
- Vitamin E
- Calcium
- Magnesium

Herbal Therapy
- Yucca
- Devil's Claw
- Boswellia
- Turmeric
- Skullcap
- Ginseng
- Bupleurum

Other
- Deep massage
- Juice Therapy (carrot, celery, cabbage, cucumber, beet)
- Massage joints with castor oil, rosemary oil, lavender oil or juniper oil

Arthritis continued

Juice Therapy

- Carrot, celery, cabbage and parsley
- Potato juice
- Cherry juice
- Carrot, beet, cucumber
- Radish, garlic
- AVOID TOMATO JUICE

AUTISM

Nutritional Therapy
- Avoid dairy products
- Avoid refined sugar
- Eliminate foods with yellow, red, and green dyes
- Eliminate monosodium glutamate (MSG)
- Eliminate aspartame

Vitamins/Minerals Therapy
- Vitamin B6
- Magnesium
- L-glutamine
- Selenium
- Omega 3's

Herbal Therapy
- Kava root

Other
- Incorporate daily structure

BAD BREATH

Nutritional Therapy
- Whole foods
- Water with fresh lemon juice
- Water with one teaspoon chlorophyll morning and night

Vitamin/Mineral Therapy
- Vitamin B Complex
- Vitamin C (1,000 mg. daily)
- Digestive enzymes
- Magnesium

Herbal Therapy
- Garlic
- Chew fennel seeds

Homeopathy
- Arnica
- Merc sol
- Nux vomica
- Kali phos

Juice Therapy
- Carrot, celery, parsley, spinach, watercress
- Wheatgrass juice
- Green juice

BACK PAIN

Vitamins/Mineral Therapy
- Glucosamine sulfate
- Glucosamine HCL
- N-acetyl-glucosamine
- Coenzyme Q10
- Vitamin C
- Vitamin E
- Calcium
- Magnesium
- Potassium

Herbal Therapy
- Willow bark
- Feverfew
- Rosemary
- Lobelia
- Yucca root
- Wild Yam

Other
- Yoga, Tai Chi, or Qigong
- Use aromatherapy, lavender, or clary sage oil

Homeopathic
- Calendula
- Arnica

<u>BED SORES</u>

Nutritional Therapy
- Distilled water
- Include plenty of fiber

Vitamin/Mineral Therapy
- Vitamin E
- Zinc
- Vitamin A
- Vitamin D

Herbal Therapy
- Garlic
- Comfrey root powder
- Echinacea powder

Homeopathy
- Calendula
- Belladonna
- Silicea

Juice Therapy
- Carrot, beet, cantaloupe currant, red grapes

Topical Therapy
- Paste of goldenseal powder
- Aloe vera gel
- Calendula cream

BERIBERI

Nutritional Therapy
- Eat brown rice and green leafy vegetables
- Eat legumes, nuts, and seeds
- Eat raw fruits
- Eat whole grains
- Do not drink with meals

Vitamin Therapy
- Thiamin (Mild- 30 mg a day divided into doses)
- Thiamin (Severe - 30-100 mg daily divided into doses)
- Vitamin B Complex

Homeopathy
- Sulfur

BLOOD CLOTS

Nutritional Therapy
- Cook with granulated garlic
- Cold water fish
- Decrease sugar intake

Vitamin Mineral Therapy
- Vitamin B6
- Niacin
- Omega-3
- Vitamin E
- Magnesium

Herbal Therapy
- Garlic capsules
- Hawthorn Berry

Homeopathy
- Hamamelis

Juice Therapy
- Garlic, carrot, parsley, spinach, celery, beet

<u>BODY ODOR</u>

Nutritional Therapy
- Whole foods
- Water with the juice of a fresh lemon and one teaspoon of chlorophyll

Vitamin/Mineral Therapy
- Vitamin B1 (50 mg two times daily while problems persist)
- Vitamin A (25,000 IU daily for a few weeks)
- Magnesium
- Chlorophyll
- Zinc

Herbal Therapy
- Dandelion
- Milk thistle

Homeopathy
- Hepar sulph
- Sulfur

Juice Therapy
- Fresh vegetable juices

BOILS

Nutritional Therapy
- Lots of green, orange, and yellow vegetables
- Water with fresh lemon juice
- Parsley

Vitamin Therapy
- Vitamin B5 (1 g four times daily)
- Coenzyme Q10
- Beta carotene
- Vitamin A

Herbal Therapy
- Echinacea
- Yellow dock
- Nettle

Homeopathy
- Belladonna
- Lachesis
- Phytolacca

Juice Therapy
- Wheatgrass
- Carrot, lettuce, spinach, yellow dock

Topical Therapy
- Hot Epsom salt pack
- Tea tree oil

BRUISES

Nutritional Therapy
- Fresh fruits
- Green leafy vegetables

Vitamin Therapy
- Vitamin C with bioflavonoids
- Vitamin B6
- Folic acid
- Vitamin E
- Iron

Herbal Therapy
- Arnica salve
- Turmeric and honey

Homeopathy
- Arnica
- Hypericum
- Hamamelis

Juice Therapy
- Carrot and beet

Topical Therapy
- Calendula ointment
- Slice of raw onion to bruise
- Witch Hazel

BUNIONS

Vitamin Therapy
- Niacinamide
- Magnesium

Herbal Therapy
- Aloe vera juice
- Parsley

Homeopathy
- Silicea
- Arnica

Reflexology Therapy
- Work around and directly on bunion

Topical Therapy
- Apply aloe vera gel

BURNS

Nutritional Therapy
- High protein diet
- Increased fluids
- Eat pumpkin seeds

Vitamin Therapy
- Vitamin E
- Vitamin C with bioflavonoids
- Vitamin A
- Vitamin B complex

Herbal Therapy
- St. John's wort
- Calendula flowers

Homeopathy
- Hypericum
- Urtica urens
- Belladonna

Juice Therapy
- Carrot, cantaloupe, currants, garlic

Topical Therapy
- Ice and vinegar

BURSITIS

Nutritional Therapy
- Eat foods high in magnesium
- Drink filtered water and apple cider vinegar
- Avoid nightshade foods

Vitamin Therapy
- Vitamin B12 (intramuscular injection)
- Calcium
- Vitamin C

Herbal Therapy
- Meadowsweet
- Horsetail
- Willow bark

Homeopathy
- Belladonna
- Arnica
- Silicea

Juice Therapy
- Equal parts carrot, celery, cucumber, beet

Topical Therapy
- Mullein hot packs - boil three to four fresh mullein leaves in water then place over joint

CANCER

Nutritional Therapy

- Avoid excessive intake of animal protein, alcohol, and caffeine
- Decrease or eliminate dairy products
- Avoid excessive intake of refined carbohydrates/sugar
- Eat broccoli daily and tomatoes daily
- Mushrooms
- Soybeans
- Omega 3 Fatty Acids
- Cook with turmeric, garlic, ginger, cayenne, sage, and rosemary

Vitamin/Mineral Therapy

- Beta carotene
- Vitamin B6
- Vitamin C
- Vitamin D
- Vitamin E
- Folic Acid
- Selenium
- Calcium/Magnesium
- Coenzyme Q10

Herbal Therapy

- Maitake Mushroom
- Astragalus
- Bromelain
- Echinacea
- Green Tea
- Green Tea

Cancer Continued
Juice Therapy
- Carrot, beet (roots and tops)
- Fresh raw cabbage and carrot juice
- Grape, black cherry, black currant
- Wheatgrass juice
- Asparagus juice
- Carrot, celery
- Carrot, spinach
- Carrot, cabbage

CANDIDIASIS

Nutritional Therapy
- Avoid sweets, alcohol and refined carbohydrates
- Remove fermented foods such as vinegar, soy sauce or pickled foods
- Olive oil
- Whole grains
- Fresh fruits
- Garlic
- Aloe Vera
- Cinnamon

Vitamin/Mineral Therapy
- Vitamin C
- Vitamin E
- Evening Primrose
- Pantothenic acid (Vitamin B5)
- Zinc chelate

Herbal Therapy
- Goldenseal
- Grapefruit seed extract
- Pau d'arco
- Oregon Grape
- Barberry
- Oil of oregano
- Tea Tree oil

CANKER SORES

Nutritional Therapy

- Eat grains
- Eat a wide variety of seeds and beans
- Avoid coffee
- Avoid alcohol
- Avoid refined food
- Avoid spicy foods

Vitamin/Mineral Therapy

- Vitamin C
- Lysine (4g for 1st four days then 500 mg 3 times daily on an empty stomach)
- Vitamin B complex
- Extra Vitamin B12
- Zinc

Herbal Therapy

- Sage mouthwash
- Echinacea

Juice Therapy

- Carrot, celery, cantaloupe

Topical Therapy

- Cotton swap each sore with 8% zinc chloride or hydrogen peroxide

CARBUNCLES

Nutritional Therapy
- Drink plenty of filtered water
- Eat whole foods with lots of green, leafy, vegetables
- Eat buckwheat

Vitamin/Mineral Therapy
- Vitamin A
- Vitamin C
- Chlorophyll
- Acidophilus

Herbal Therapy
- Refer to boils

Homeopathy
- Ledum
- Belladonna
- Arsen alb

Juice Therapy
- Carrot, beet, celery and garlic
- Wheatgrass and cucumber

Topical Therapy
- Refer to boils

CARPAL TUNNEL SYNDROME

Nutritional Therapy
- Whole foods diet
- Limit protein intake
- Eliminate foods high in yellow dyes
- Eat whole grains, seeds, nuts
- Eat fresh salmon
- Avoid sugar, caffeine, and processed corn

Vitamin/Mineral Therapy
- Vitamin B6 (highly effective)
- Vitamin B Complex
- Magnesium
- Essential Fatty Acids
- Folic Acid
- Bromelain

Herbal Therapy
- Meadowsweet
- Willow Bark
- Butcher's Broom
- Devil's Claw
- Cayenne

Lifestyle Therapy
- Avoid repetitive wrist movement

CELLULITE

Nutritional Therapy
- Whole foods
- Less complex carbohydrates
- Do not eat proteins at night

Herbal Therapy
- Horse chestnut bark
- Gotu kola

Body Therapy
- Massage the affected area regularly

Juice Therapy
- Beet, carrot

Topical Therapy
- Aloe vera extract

CEREBRAL PALSY

Nutritional Therapy
- Get tested for food allergies

Vitamin/Mineral Therapy
- Magnesium
- Vitamin B1
- Vitamin B6
- Vitamin C

CHEMICAL POISONING

Nutritional Therapy
- Eat organically grown foods
- Fast regularly
- Eat a high fiber diet
- Eat brown rice, barley, oatmeal
- Eat beets, carrots, spinach, bananas

Vitamin/Mineral Therapy
- Vitamin C (3,000mg daily for a week)
- Vitamin B complex
- Vitamin E
- Selenium
- L-Cysteine
- Garlic capsules

Herbal Therapy
- Milk thistle
- Licorice
- Dandelion

CHRONIC FATIGUE SYNDROME

Nutritional Therapy
- Complex carbohydrates - vegetables, grains, beans
- Avoid foods high in sugar

Vitamin/Mineral Therapy
- Beta carotene
- Vitamin C
- Pantothenic acid
- Zinc
- B Vitamins
- Magnesium

Herbal Therapy
- Echinacea
- Goldenseal
- Licorice
- Siberian Ginseng
- Nettle
- Noni

Juice Therapy
- Wheatgrass juice

CHRONIC PAIN

Nutritional Therapy
- Detoxify by fasting once a week
- Limit caffeine and alcohol
- Avoid excessive consumption of red meats and dairy products

Vitamin/Mineral Therapy
- Vitamin C
- Evening primrose oil
- Vitamin E
- Magnesium

Herbal Therapy
- Devil's Claw

Other

- Hydrotherapy
- Aromatherapy - marjoram, clary sage, ginger, birch

<u>CIRRHOSIS</u>

Nutritional Therapy
- Eat whole foods including nuts, seeds, beans
- Eat a low protein diet
- Avoid dairy products
- Use cold-processed oils

Vitamin/Mineral Therapy
- Vitamin B complex
- Vitamin B12
- Folic acid
- Vitamin C
- L-carnitine
- L-cysteine

Herbal Therapy
- Milk thistle (70 - 200 mg daily)
- Licorice

Juice Therapy
- Beet and carrot
- Wheat grass
- Add raw flaxseed oil and garlic to juices

Aromatherapy
- Juniper
- Rosemary
- Rose

COLDS AND FLU

Nutritional Therapy
- NONE - starve a cold
- Green and orange vegetables for prevention and recovery

Vitamins/Minerals Therapy
- Vitamin C
- Vitamin A
- Zinc
- N-Acetyl-Cysteine
- Selenium

Herbal Therapy
- Yarrow
- Eyebright
- Elecampane
- Elderflower
- Mullein

Homeopathy
- Aconitum napellus
- Natrum muriaticum
- Allium cepa
- Nux Vomica
- Eupatorium perfoliatum

Other

- Adequate sleep

Colds Continued
Colds and flu continued

- Inhalations and baths with camphor, eucalyptus, lemon, peppermint, pine, rosemary and tea tree oil.

Juice Therapy

- Lemon, orange, pineapple, black currant, elderberry juice
- Carrot, beet, tomato, green pepper, watercress
- Carrot, spinach
- Add small doses of ginger, onion or garlic to all juices

COLD SORES (HERPES SIMPLEX)

Nutritional Therapy
- Eat more raw vegetables

Vitamin/Mineral Therapy
- L-lysine (4g daily for the first four days then 500 mg three times daily)
- Vitamin B complex
- Vitamin C
- Zinc gluconate
- Vitamin E
- Quercetin

Herbal Therapy
- Echinacea
- Siberian ginseng
- Nettle
- Goldenseal

Aromatherapy
- Geranium
-
- Lemon
- Chamomile
- Tea tree
- Lavender

Juice Therapy
- Avoid citrus and pineapple

CONVULSIONS

Nutritional Therapy
- Eat small meals
- Avoid caffeine
- Avoid aspartame

Vitamin/Mineral Therapy
- Vitamin B6
- Manganese
- Folic Acid
- Vitamin B3
- Vitamin D
- Copper
- Magnesium
- Selenium

Herbal Therapy
- Asafetida
- Mugwort
- Skullcap
- Valerian root

Homeopathy
- Cuprum met
- Belladonna

Aromatherapy
- Chamomile
- Clary

<u>CORNS</u>

Nutritional Therapy
- Whole foods diet

Vitamin/Mineral Therapy
- Vitamin A
- Vitamin E
- Essential Fatty Acids

Homeopathy
- Graphites
- Silicea
- Antim crud

Massage Therapy
- Massage around and directly on the corns

Topical Therapy
- Aloe vera gel
- Rub castor oil on corn twice daily

COUGHS

Nutritional Therapy
- Eat whole foods including lots of raw fruits and vegetables
- Avoid mucus-producing foods
- Drink pineapple juice
- Eat honey

Vitamin/Mineral Therapy
- Zinc
- Vitamin A
- Vitamin C

Herbal Therapy
- Coltsfoot
- Mullein
- Marshmallow

Homeopathy
- Belladonna
- Aconite
- Bryonia
- Kali bich
- Ipecac

Juice Therapy
- Fresh fruit and vegetable juices
- Hot pear juice with cinnamon stick

DANDRUFF

Nutritional Therapy

- Increase raw foods
- Eat salads daily
- Avoid fried foods
- Avoid seafood
- Avoid sugar
- Avoid nuts

Vitamin/Mineral Therapy

- Vitamin B Complex
- Vitamin A
- Omega-6
- Vitamin C
- Kelp tablets

Herbal Therapy

- Rinse hair with nettle, sage, and rosemary mixture
- Evening Primrose (3 capsules daily)

Homeopathy

- Arsen alb
- Graphites
- Lycopodium
- Thuja

Alternative Therapy

- Do hot Apple Cider Vinegar hair treatment, rinse

DERMATITIS

Nutritional Therapy
- Avoid dairy
- Eat naturally fermented foods

Vitamin/Mineral Therapy
- Vitamin B Complex
- Omega-6 Fatty Acids
- Zinc
- Magnesium

Herbal Therapy
- Nettle
- Red Clover

Homeopathy
- Pulsatilla
- Arsen alb
- Sulfur
- Sepia

Juice Therapy
- Carrot, beet, cucumber, celery
- Carrot, celery, apple
- Cantaloupe

DIABETES

Nutritional Therapy

- Eliminate refined sugar and sugar products
- Avoid junk foods
- Eat whole grains, fresh vegetables, and fresh fruits
- Reduce or eliminate alcohol, tobacco, and caffeine intake

Vitamins/Minerals Therapy

- B-complex vitamins
- Chromium
- Magnesium
- EFA's
- Vitamin C
- Coenzyme Q10

Herbal Therapy

- Fenugreek
- Garlic
- Ginseng
- Bitter melon
- Neem

Other

- Oxygen Therapy

Juice Therapy

- String beans, parsley, cucumber, watercress
- Carrot, celery, parsley, spinach

DIZZINESS

Nutritional Therapy
- Eat small meals throughout the day
- Avoid caffeinated beverages
- Avoid alcohol

Vitamin/Mineral Therapy
- Niacin
- Vitamin E
- Iron

Herbal Therapy
- Ginger
- Ginkgo Leaf Extract

Homeopathy
- Gelsemium
- Phosphorus
- Cocculus
- Granatum

DYSENTERY

Nutritional Therapy
- Clove of garlic morning and evening
- Avoid alcohol

Vitamin/Mineral Therapy
- Acidophilus
- Vitamin A
- Citrus seed extract

Herbal Therapy
- Oak bark
- Chamomile
- Use electrolyte replacement

ECZEMA

Nutritional Therapy
- Avoid wheat
- Avoid dairy
- Avoid citrus fruits during outbreaks

Vitamin/Mineral Therapy
- Zinc
- Vitamin A
- GLA (gamma-linolenic acid)
- Evening Primrose Oil
- Vitamin B Complex

Herbal Therapy
- Cleavers
- Nettle
- Yellow Dock

Homeopathy
- Dulcamara
- Rhus tox
- Sulfur

Juice Therapy
- Black currant, red grapes
- Carrot, beet, spinach, cucumber, parsley
- Wheat grass

Topical Therapy
- Apply Evening Primrose Oil

EDEMA

Nutritional Therapy
- Avoid caffeine
- Avoid alcohol
- Avoid dairy products
- Avoid white flour
- Avoid chocolate
- Avoid olives
- Avoid pickles
- Avoid soy sauce

Vitamin/Mineral Therapy
- Vitamin B Complex
- Potassium
- Vitamin C
- Alfalfa Tablets

Herbal Therapy
- Dandelion
- Horse Chestnut Seed

Juice Therapy
- Pears, pineapple, watermelon, cranberries
- Green juices (add a bit of dandelion juice)
- Cucumber, parsley, celery, carrot

EPILEPSY

Nutritional Therapy
- Low fat, low carbohydrate diet
- Eliminate fried foods
- Avoid milk
- Avoid alcohol
- Avoid caffeine

Vitamin/Mineral Therapy
- L-tyrosine (500 mg three times daily)
- Vitamin B Complex
- Manganese
- Zinc
- Choline (start with 4 g daily, increase to 10 g daily after 3 months)
- Intramuscular B Complex may be helpful

Herbal Therapy
- Skullcap Tincture

Juice Therapy
- Celery, carrot, and lettuce juice three times daily

FIBROMYALGIA

Nutritional Therapy
- Vegetarian Diet

Vitamins/Minerals Therapy
- Vitamin B3
- Vitamin C
- Vitamin E
- EFA's
- Selenium
- Zinc

Herbal Therapy
- Cayenne
- Chamomile

Homeopathy
- Arnica
- Bryonia

Other
- Lavender oil
- Rosemary oil
- Clary sage oil

FLATULENCE

Nutritional Therapy
- Do not overeat
- Chew food slowly and thoroughly
- Consume high fiber foods

Vitamin/Mineral Therapy
- Vitamin B Complex
- Hydrochloric Acid
- Charcoal Tablets

Herbal Therapy
- Anise

Homeopathy
- Carbo veg
- Lycopodium
- Nux mosch.

Juice Therapy
- Papaya Juice
- Carrot, parsley, beet, celery

Other Therapy
- Drink water with several drops of peppermint oil throughout the day
- Rub abdomen in clockwise direction

FOOD POISONING

Nutritional Therapy
- Stop eating solid foods until better
- Drink plenty of fluids
- Only drink bottled water

Vitamin/Mineral Therapy
- Acidophilus
- Charcoal tablets (6 tablets immediately upon being poisoned)
- Citrus seed extract
- Garlic capsule
- Vitamin C with bioflavonoids

Homeopathy
- Arsen alb.
- Chamomilla
- Ipecac
- Apis mel.
- Nux vom

Juice Therapy
- Carrot, beet, garlic

FRACTURES

Nutritional Therapy
- Dark leafy greens
- Raw seeds and nuts
- Avoid excessive consumption of caffeine
- Avoid red meat
- Avoid processed foods

Vitamin/Mineral Therapy
- Calcium
- Magnesium
- Vitamin C with bioflavonoids
- Vitamin D
- Vitamin K

Herbal Therapy
- Comfrey leaf
- Horsetail

Homeopathy
- Calc phos.
- Symphytum
- Ruta grav.
- Arnica

Juice Therapy
- Add watercress to beet and carrot juice

FUNGAL INFECTION

Nutritional Therapy
- Whole foods diet
- Avoid foods high in yeast, i.e, beer, bread
- Avoid sugar

Vitamin/Mineral Therapy
- Acidophilus
- Garlic capsules
- Vitamin B Complex
- Pantothenic Acid
- Vitamin C
- Vitamin E

Herbal Therapy
- Myrrh
- Tea Tree Oil

Homeopathy
- Calendula
- Chamomilla
- Belladonna
- Sulfur

Juice Therapy
- Avoid fruit juices
- Add garlic to vegetable juices

GALL BLADDER DISORDERS

Nutritional Therapy
- Whole food diet
- No animal products
- No processed foods
- Drink fresh apple juice
- Eat apples
- Drink ½ cup olive oil mixed with ⅓ cup fresh lemon juice

Vitamin/Mineral Therapy
- Vitamin C
- Vitamin B Complex
- Choline
- Alfalfa Tablets
- Lecithin

Herbal Therapy
- Wild Yam
- Fringetree Bark
- Milk Thistle

Juice Therapy
- Carrot, beet, cucumber (add a little garlic, radish or fresh dandelion root)
- Grape, pear, grapefruit, lemon

GASTROINTESTINAL DISORDERS

Nutritional Therapy

- Plenty of fresh, organic fruits and vegetables
- Fiber-rich foods
- Avoid processed foods
- Avoid food additives, preservatives, sugar, caffeine, and alcohol

Vitamins/Minerals Therapy

- Probiotics
- Hydrochloric acid

Homeopathy

- Aloe
- Allium sativa
- Belladonna
- Nux Vomica

Other

- Regular exercise
- Reflexology
- Hydrogen peroxide therapy

Juice Therapy

- Cabbage, papaya, carrot
- Wheatgrass juice
- Raw potato juice
- AVOID CITRUS JUICE

HAIR LOSS

Nutritional Therapy
- Whole food diets with foods with skin i.e, potato skins, cucumbers
- Len meats
- Raisins
- Sea vegetables

Vitamin/Mineral Therapy
- Flaxseed Oil
- Biotin
- Zinc
- Trace minerals
- Iron

Herbal Therapy
- Massage scalp with rosemary and almond oil

Homeopathy
- Sepia
- Arnica
- Acidum nit.

Juice Therapy
- Carrot, beet, spinach, nettle, alfalfa
- Add onion juice to vegetable juice

HANGOVER

Nutritional Therapy
- Eat dry whole grain bread before drinking
- Drink water with 1 tsp. Turmeric before and after drinking
- Drink tomato juice the morning after
- Drink water with lemon juice

Vitamin/Mineral Therapy
- Vitamin B Complex
- Vitamin C
- Folic Acid

Herbal Therapy
- Dandelion Root
- Mugwort
- Gentian
- Milk Thistle
- Activated charcoal

Homeopathy
- Nux vom.
- Arsen alb.
- Aconite
- Sulfur

Juice Therapy
- Turmeric, lemon, tomato

HEADACHES

Nutritional Therapy

- Get tested for food allergies

Vitamins/Minerals Therapy

- Vitamin C
- Vitamin E
- Vitamin B3
- Calcium
- Magnesium

Herbal Therapy

- Feverfew
- Ginkgo biloba

Aromatherapy (massaged into temples)

- Lavender
- Peppermint
- Rosemary
- Eucalyptus
- Chamomile

Juice Therapy

- Carrot, celery
- Carrot, beet, cucumber
- Carrot, celery, spinach, parsley

HEARING AND EAR DISORDERS

Nutritional Therapy
- Reduce saturated fats
- Limit wheat intake
- Limit dairy intake
- Reduce sugar and alcohol intake

Vitamins/Minerals Therapy
- Beta carotene
- Vitamin C
- Vitamin E
- N-acetyl-cysteine
- Folic acid

Herbal Therapy
- Ginkgo biloba
- Black cohosh
- Goldenseal
- Mullein
- St. John's wort

Other
- Use tea tree oil drops and diluted grapefruit seed extract for ringing in the ears, diminished hearing, ear pain, or ear problems caused by yeast infections

Homeopathic Therapy
- Belladonna
- Apis mellifica
- Aconitum napellus

Hearing and ear disorders continued
- Lachesis
- Lycopodium

HEART DISEASE

Nutritional Therapy

- Foods free of pesticides, herbicides, steroids and antibiotics
- Increase fiber intake from green leafy vegetables & fresh raw fruits
- Use olive oils
- Avoid fried foods
- Limit animal fats
- Eliminate sugar, tobacco, and alcohol

Vitamins/Minerals Therapy

- Beta carotene
- Vitamin B3
- Vitamin B12
- Folic acid
- Calcium
- Chromium
- Selenium
- Coenzyme Q10

Herbal Therapy

- Foxglove
- Hawthorn berry
- Garlic
- Ginger
- Motherwort

Juice Therapy

- Carrot, celery, cucumber, beet, garlic or hawthorn berry
- Blueberries, blackberries, black currant, red grapes

HEMORRHOIDS

Nutritional Therapy
- Whole foods with an emphasis on high-fiber foods
- Citrus fruits
- Drink plenty of fluids
- One tablespoon of olive or coconut oil (with food or alone)

Vitamin/Mineral Therapy
- Vitamin C with Bioflavonoids (3-6 g. daily)
- Vitamin A (10,000-25,000 IU daily)
- Folic Acid (400-800 mcg)
- Vitamin B Complex (two times daily)
- Essential Fatty Acids (three to four on empty stomach)
- Magnesium
- Zinc

Herbal Therapy
- St. John's Salve
- Calendula
- Butcher's Broom
- Comfrey Root
- Gotu Kola
- Horse Chestnut
- Parsley
- Passionflower

Homeopathy
- Aloe
- Nux Vom

HEPATITIS

Nutritional Therapy
- Low protein
- Avoid sugar
- Avoid caffeine
- Avoid alcohol
- Drink fresh lemon juice

Vitamin/Mineral Therapy
- Vitamin C
- Beta Carotene (100,000 IU daily for 2 weeks then reduce to 25,000-50,000 IU)
- Vitamin B Complex
- Pantothenic Acid
- Beta Hydrochloric Acid

Herbal Therapy
- Milk Thistle
- Dandelion Root
- Licorice

Juice Therapy
- Short juice fast using beet, carrot and wheatgrass juices
- Garlic, burdock, flax, black currants

HIATAL HERNIA

Nutritional Therapy

- Avoid overeating
- Avoid eating spicy foods
- Avoid eating fried foods
- Avoid coffee, tea, and carbonated drinks
- Avoid eating onions, and red or green peppers
- Avoid peppermint
- Eat plenty of fiber

Vitamin/Mineral Therapy

- Digestive enzymes
- Vitamin B Complex
- Chlorophyll (at dinner time for one week)
- Mineral formula

Herbal Therapy

- Comfrey root
- Marshmallow root
- Meadowsweet

Homeopathy

- Calc carb
- Hepar sulph
- Ferrum Phos

HICCUPS

Nutritional Therapy
- Chew dry toast
- Slowly sip glass of water while walking continuously
- Eat papaya

Vitamin/Mineral Therapy
- Papaya enzymes
- Digestive enzymes

Herbal Therapy
- Black cohosh
- Skullcap
- Vervain

Homeopathy
- Nux vom
- Mag Phos
- Ignatia
- Lycopodium
- Ginseng
- Acidum sulf

Juice Therapy
- Swish juice in mouth before swallowing

HIVES

Nutritional Therapy
- Avoid berries
- Avoid fish
- Avoid soy
- Avoid citrus
- Avoid peanuts

Vitamin/Mineral Therapy
- Pancreatic enzymes (4 times daily on empty stomach during initial attack)
- Bromelain
- Vitamin C
- Vitamin B Complex (2 -4 times daily with lots of water then reduce to 2 times daily after two days)
- Sodium bicarbonate ($\frac{1}{2}$ tsp dissolved in water on empty stomach and 30 minutes before eating another meal)
- Essential Fatty Acids

Herbal Therapy
- Parsley
- Peppermint Oil

Homeopathy
- Apis mel
- Nat mur
- Urtica urens

HYPERTENSION

Nutritional Therapy
- Reduce your weight
- Eliminate salt
- Avoid alcohol
- Increase potassium in your diet
- Eat more celery, garlic, and onions

Vitamins/Minerals Therapy
- Calcium
- Magnesium
- Vitamin C
- Zinc
- Flaxseed oil

Herbal Therapy
- Hawthorn berry

Juice Therapy
- Celery, beet, and carrot or cucumber, spinach and parsley

Aromatherapy
- Ylang ylang
- Marjoram
- Lavender

HYPERTHYROIDISM

Nutritional Therapy
- Foods that naturally and gently suppress thyroid hormone production such as:
- Eat broccoli
- Eat brussel sprouts
- Eat cabbage
- Eat kale
- Eat spinach
- Eat mustard greens
- Eat peaches
- Avoid dairy products
- Avoid caffeinated products

Vitamin/Mineral Therapy
- Vitamin A
- Choline
- Vitamin B complex (with extra thiamin)
- Amino acids
- Kelp
- Magnesium and calcium

Juice Therapy
- Carrot, celery, spinach, parsley
- Cabbage, watercress, and spinach

HYPOGLYCEMIA

Nutritional Therapy

- Smaller, more frequent meals
- Avoid caffeine
- Avoid alcohol
- Focus on whole grains, seeds, nuts
- Avoid dairy products
- Avoid processed foods
- Avoid white flour products
- Eat lean meats
- Eat high amounts of fiber

Vitamin/Mineral Therapy

- Chromium (100 mcg three times daily)
- Niacinamide
- Pantothenic acid
- Vitamin C with bioflavonoids
- Vitamin B Complex

Herbal Therapy

- Licorice
- Burdock
- Dandelion

Juice Therapy

- Dilute all juices
- Carrot, beet with burdock, Jerusalem artichoke, garlic

HYPOTHYROIDISM

Nutritional Therapy
- Foods high in iodine such as fish, kelp, vegetables, root vegetables
- Avoid foods that naturally slow the functioning of the thyroid such as:
- Avoid cabbage
- Avoid brussel sprouts
- Avoid mustard greens
- Avoid broccoli
- Avoid turnips
- Avoid kale
- Avoid spinach
- Avoid peaches

Vitamin/Mineral Therapy
- Calcium/magnesium
- Vitamin B Complex
- Tyrosine
- Iodine
- Essential Fatty Acids
- Vitamin A
- Zinc
- Kelp

Herbal Therapy
- Gentian
- Mugwort
- Cascara sagrada
- St. John's Wort

INFECTION

Nutritional Therapy

- Use large amounts of dietary garlic
- Drink large amounts of orange juice, apple juice, cranberries, strawberries
- Eat raw honey
- Drink plenty of filtered water

Vitamin/Mineral Therapy

- Vitamin A (400,000 IU daily for five days)
- Garlic extract (liquid or capsules, doubled bottle dosage)
- Essential Fatty Acids

Herbal Therapy

- Echinacea
- Goldenseal
- Oregon Grape
- Siberian Ginseng
- Grapefruit Seed Extract

Juice Therapy

- Water only fast for 24-48 hours
- Carrot, celery, beet, cantaloupe

INFLAMMATION

Nutritional Therapy
- 75% raw foods diet
- Avoid white sugar and white flour
- Drink water with 1 tsp lemon juice

Vitamin/Mineral Therapy
- Vitamin C with bioflavonoids (3 g the first hour, then 1 g every two hours for the first few days, then 3g per day)
- Zinc (30-60 mg daily)
- Beta carotene (100,000 IU first three days then reduce to 25,000 IU for several weeks)
- Primrose oil
- Vitamin A and E emulsion
- Calcium
- Mineral formula

Herbal Therapy
- Digestive inflammation - chamomile, lemon balm, licorice or meadowsweet
- Skin inflammation - calendula, St. John's Wort, plantain
- Rheumatic or Arthritic inflammation - willow bark, meadowsweet or wild yam, sea cucumber, yarrow

Homeopathy
- Belladonna
- Ferrum phos
- Sulfur

INSECT BITES

Vitamin/Mineral Therapy

- Vitamin C as soon as possible (5g) with B5 (1g) continue taking 1 g of vitamin c and 500 mg of B's every hour until pain and swelling subside
- Vitamin E (apply to sting)

Herbal Therapy

- Apply aloe gel

Homeopathy

- Aconite
- Lachesis
- Apil mel
- Hypercium
- Urtica urens
- Calendula

JAUNDICE

Nutritional Therapy
- Eat raw foods
- Eat fruits and vegetables
- Glass of warm water with lemon juice upon rising
- Eat plenty of green vegetables and sprouts to cleanse the blood

Vitamin/Mineral Therapy
- Digestive enzymes
- Vitamin C
- Vitamin B Complex
- Protein Supplements

Herbal Therapy
- Chickweed
- Dandelion
- Gentian Root
- Goldenseal
- Parsley
- Rose
- Yellow Dock

Homeopathy
- Bryonia
- Chelidonium
- Nux vom

Juice Therapy
- Carrot, beet, cucumber

KIDNEY STONES

Nutritional Therapy

- Increase fluids
- Increase fiber and green vegetables
- Avoid refined sugar
- Drink at least eight glasses of water or more daily
- Eat cranberries
- Eat black cherries
- Drink kombucha tea

Vitamin/Mineral Therapy

- Magnesium (200 mg two times daily)
- Vitamin B6 (50 mg three times daily)
- Vitamin C
- Fat soluble chlorophyll

Herbal Therapy

- Cornsilk
- Wild Yam
- Blackhaw
- Uva Ursi
- Horsetail
- Dandelion

Juice Therapy

- Lemon juice
- Carrot, beet, and cucumber juice (add a little garlic)
- Cranberry, watermelon

LARYNGITIS

Nutritional Therapy
- Whole foods
- Plenty of fluids
- Avoid refined carbohydrates

Vitamin/Mineral Therapy
- Vitamin A (100,000 IU for first three days)
- Vitamin C
- Garlic Capsules

Herbal Therapy
- Red sage
- Yarrow
- Chamomile
- Echinacea extract (30 drops every hour for 2 days)
- Gargle with sage

Homeopathy
- Aconite
- Hepar sulph
- Phosphorus
- Belladonna
- Kali bich

Juice Therapy
- Carrot, pineapple
- Carrot, apple
- Carrot, beet, cucumber, ginger

LUPUS

Nutritional Therapy
- Whole foods
- Small meals
- Avoid cow's milk
- Avoid beef products
- Increase yellow, green, & orange vegetables
- Avoid alfalfa sprouts

Vitamin/Mineral Therapy
- Vitamin C with bioflavonoids
- Digestive enzymes with meals
- Calcium/Magnesium
- Essential Fatty Acids
- L-cysteine
- L-methionine
- Beta Carotene
- Vitamin E (1,500 IU daily)
- Garlic
- Vitamin B Complex

Herbal Therapy
- Licorice
- Wild yam
- Nettle
- Echinacea
- Pau d'arco

Juice Therapy
- Carrot, celery, flaxseed oil,garlic

LYME DISEASE

Nutritional Therapy
- Avoid alcohol
- Avoid sugars
- Mineral formula
- Increase alkaline food intake (green vegetables, complex grains, almonds, uams, lentils, squash)

Vitamin/Mineral Therapy
- Borage oil
- Coenzyme Q10
- Calcium pantothenate (500 mg three times daily)
- Biotin (650 mg 2-3 times daily)
- L-Carnitine
- Magnesium

Herbal Therapy (under the guidance of a professional)
- Astragalus
- Ginseng
- Maitake mushrooms
- Reishi mushrooms
- Cordyceps

MEMORY AND COGNITION PROBLEMS

Nutritional Therapy
- Whole foods
- Fish
- Nuts
- Seeds

Vitamin/Mineral Therapy
- Super Choline
- Pantothenic acid
- Vitamin B Complex
- Lecithin
- DMAE (dimethylaminoethanol)

Herbal Therapy
- Ginkgo biloba
- Siberian Ginseng
- Ashwagandha
- Bilberry
- Garlic
- Green Tea
- Kelp
- Peppermint Leaf
- Rosemary
- Gotu kola
- skullcap

Homeopathy
- Arsen alb.

MENTAL HEALTH

Nutritional Therapy
- Eat a variety of foods
- Don't overeat or binge
- Avoid foods with dyes
- Avoid processed foods

Vitamins/Minerals Therapy
- Vitamin B1, B3, B6, B12
- Vitamin C
- Sodium
- Potassium
- Manganese
- Zinc

Herbal Therapy
- St. John's Wort

Juice Therapy
- Seasonal fruit and vegetable juices

Aromatherapy
- Chamomile
- Lavender
- Sandalwood
- Bergamot
- Neroli

MONONUCLEOSIS

Nutritional Therapy
- Drink plenty of water
- Avoid animal intake
- Drink vegetable protein drinks
- Eat small meals
- Eat vegetable soups
- Avoid processed and fried foods

Vitamin/Mineral Therapy
- Vitamin C to bowel tolerance
- Vitamin A (50,000 IU daily for 2 months)
- Vitamin E (400 -6-- IU daily)
- Vitamin B Complex (low dose, three to four times daily)
- Chlorophyll

Herbal Therapy
- Myrrh
- Echinacea
- Wormwood
- Calendula

Homeopathy
- Belladonna
- Merc iod
- Phytolacca

Juice Therapy
- Carrot, beet, tomato, green pepper

MOTION SICKNESS

Nutritional Therapy
- Avoid eating or drinking large amounts
- Sip small amounts of fresh lemon or lime juice
- Drink ginger tea
- Drink green tea

Vitamin/Mineral Therapy
- Ginger (4 capsules taken 2 hours before travel and 1 per hour for the first few hours of travel)
- Vitamin B Complex
- Vitamin B6 (50 mg)
- Magnesium (100 mg)
- Charcoal tablets (4 taken several hours before travel if ginger has proven not effective in past)

Homeopathy
- Ipecac
- Colchicum
- Nux vom
- Ignatia
- Belladonna

Juice Therapy
- Any combination with ginger added

MULTIPLE SCLEROSIS

Nutritional Therapy
- Get tested for food allergies
- Avoid dairy and caffeine
- Avoid wheat gluten
- Adopt a low fat diet
- Avoid monosodium glutamate (MSG)
- Eat tofu, bean sprouts, nuts and seeds

Vitamins/Minerals Therapy
- Omega-3 fatty acids
- Vitamins B1, B3, B6, B12
- Vitamin C
- Zinc
- Magnesium
- Selenium
- Alpha-lipoic acid

Juice Therapy
- Short fasts with fruit and vegetable juices

Aromatherapy
- Rub affected parts with a mixture of 95% olive oil and 5% essence of juniper or rosemary

Other
- Avoid chemical pollution

MUSCULAR CRAMPS

Nutritional Therapy
- Whole foods diet
- Leafy green vegetables
- Apricots
- Sesame seeds
- alfalfa

Vitamin/Mineral Therapy
- Magnesium aspartate
- Calcium
- Vitamin E (400 IU three times daily)
- Vitamin B Complex with extra niacin (B6)
- Vitamin C
- Chlorophyll
- Folic acid (500 mcg three times daily)

Herbal Therapy
- Cramp bark tea
- Lobelia

Juice Therapy
- Carrot, beet, celery, cucumber
- Sweet fruit juices

NAUSEA

Nutritional Therapy

- Eat small meals
- Avoid fats
- Sip lemon water
- Avoid MSG
- Avoid aspartame (Nutrasweet)

Vitamin/Mineral Therapy

- Vitamin B Complex
- Vitamin B6
- Magnesium

Herbal Therapy

- Ginger
- Peppermint

Homeopathy

- Ipecac
- Nux Vom
- Pulsatilla
- Calc fluor
- Colchicum

NOSEBLEEDS

Nutritional Therapy
- Watercress
- Dark green leafy vegetables
- Kale
- Alfalfa

Vitamin/Mineral Therapy
- Vitamin C (3 g at start and 1 g every hour if bleeding continues)

Herbal Therapy
- Oak bark

Homeopathy
- Hyoscyamus
- Chamomilla
- Rhus tox
- Ipecac
- Belladonna

Juice Therapy
- Carrot, beet with ginger or cayenne

Other Therapy
- Place a bit of cayenne pepper on tongue
- Sit down and place head tipped forward

OSTEOPOROSIS

Nutritional Therapy

- Leafy green vegetables
- Whole grains
- Red meat less than twice per week
- Avoid soft drinks
- Limit alcohol consumption
- Remove salt from diet

Vitamins/Minerals Therapy

- Vitamin D
- Vitamin C
- Beta carotene
- Calcium
- Vitamin B6
- Vitamin K
- Magnesium
- Manganese
- Hydrochloric acid

Juice Therapy

- Green Juice
- Beet, carrot, and celery
- Lemon, papaya, pineapple

Ayurvedic Medicine

- 1 part sesame seeds, half part giner, with raw sugar added to taste. Eat teaspoon daily.

Herbal Medicine

- Horsetail
- Dandelion

PANCREATITIS

Nutritional Therapy
- For acute cases, fast from all foods and liquids
- Avoid refined sugars
- Avoid caffeine
- Avoid alcohol
- Eat small frequent meals
- Limit fruit intake
- Eat large amounts of vegetables

Vitamin/Mineral Therapy
- Chromium (300 mcg daily)
- Vitamin B Complex with extra niacin
- Vitamin C buffered
- Magnesium
- Liquid chlorophyll

Herbal Therapy
- Fringetree bark
- Balmony
- Milk Thistle

Juice Therapy
- Carrot, Jerusalem artichoke
- Beet, and garlic diluted with water

PARALYSIS

Nutritional Therapy
- Whole foods diet
- Dark leafy greens
- Green drinks
- Avoid excessive consumption of refined sugars
- Avoid caffeinated beverages

Vitamin/Mineral Therapy
- Vitamin B6
- Magnesium
- Niacinamide
- Vitamin B Complex
- Vitamin C

Homeopathy
- Aconite
- Arsen alb
- Ignatia
- Chamomilla
- Colchicum
- Conium mac

PARASITIC INFECTIONS

Nutritional Therapy

- Cook meats to well done
- Eliminate sugar
- Eliminate dairy products
- Eat pineapple
- Eat papaya
- Eat onions
- Eat ground almonds
- Eat blackberries

Herbal Therapy

- Citrus seed extract

Ayurvedic Medicine

- Indian long pepper
- Triphala

Aromatherapy

- Bergamot
- Chamomile
- Camphor
- Lavender
- Peppermint

Other

- Apply tea tree or thyme oil for skin infections

PARKINSON'S DISEASE

Nutritional Therapy
- Whole foods diet (at least 75% of diet)
- Lots of fluids
- Eat sesame seeds
- Eat rutabagas
- Eat sprouts

Vitamin/Mineral Therapy
- GABA (500 mg once daily)
- Calcium/Magnesium
- Lecithin
- Vitamin C
- Vitamin E (1,000 IU daily)

Herbal Therapy
- Passionflower

Juice Therapy
- Carrot and spinach
- Carrot, radish, garlic, and cucumber

PELLAGRA

Nutritional Therapy
- Whole grains
- Bananas
- Raw seeds and nuts
- Liver
- Avocados
- Broccoli
- Tomatoes
- Collard greens

Vitamin/Mineral Therapy
- Niacinamide (300 - 1,000 mg in divided doses, three times daily)
- Vitamin B Complex (100 mg. Three times daily)
- Protein supplements

Other Therapy
- Magnetic therapy
- Traditional Chinese Medicine

PERIODONTAL (GUM) DISEASE

Nutritional Therapy
- Eat fresh fruits
- Eat fresh vegetables (5-7 servings daily)
- Avoid refined sugars
- Avoid carbohydrates
- Drink sufficient water
- Eat blueberries
- Eat grapes

Vitamin/Mineral Therapy
- Folic acid (500 mcg to 1 mg daily)
- Vitamin C (1 - 3g daily) with bioflavonoids
- Vitamin A (25,000 IU daily for several months)
- Calcium (650-1.500 mg daily)
- Vitamin B Complex
- Beta Carotene
- Vitamin K
- Zinc

Herbal Therapy
- Sage
- Chamomile
- Echinacea

Juice Therapy
- Carrot and cantaloupe

PLEURISY

Nutritional Therapy
- Eat fresh fruits
- Eat vegetables
- Eat hearty soups
- Use turmeric generously

Vitamin/Mineral Therapy
- Vitamin A (200,000 IU first three days, reduce to 100,000 next three days, then 50,000 for IU for next two weeks)
- Vitamin C with bioflavonoids
- Essential Fatty Acids
- Bromelain (100 - 200 mg daily)

Herbal Therapy
- Mullein
- Pleurisy
- Garlic capsule

Homeopathy
- Aconite
- Bryonia
- Apis mel
- Cantharis
- Kali carb

Juice Therapy
- Carrot, celery, parsley
- Carrot, pineapple

POISON OAK/IVY

Vitamin/Mineral Therapy

- Vitamin C (3g first hour, then 1 g per hour for few days)
- Vitamin A (100,000 IU first two days in severe cases. 50,000 if less severe. Then reduce to 25,000 IU for three days)
- Vitamin E (1,000 IU for first several days)
- Vitamin B Complex

Herbal Therapy

- Mugwort
- White oak bark

Topical Therapy

- Rinse affected area with apple cider vinegar and goldenseal
- Apply aloe vera gel and/or baking soda paste (baking soda mixed with water)
- Apply activated charcoal paste (open a capsule of activated charcoal, mix with water or witch hazel and apply)

<u>POLIO</u>

Nutritional Therapy
- Whole foods diet
- Dark green leafy vegetables

Vitamin/Mineral Therapy
- Magnesium (100 - 800 mg daily to stool tolerance. Once bowels are very soft, decrease to 100 - 200 mg daily)
- Niacinamide (4 times daily, taken regularly for effectiveness)

Juice Therapy
- Carrot, beet, radish, celery

PSORIASIS

Nutritional Therapy

- Eat a varied diet rotating foods
- Eliminate wheat
- Eat seafood
- Eat olive oil
- Eat flaxseed

Vitamin/Mineral Therapy

- Vitamin A (75,000 IU daily for first two weeks, then reduce to 50,000 IU daily for two to three months)
- Folic Acid (100-500 mcg daily)
- Vitamin B Complex
- Lecithin

Herbal Therapy

- Sarsaparilla
- Burdock
- Cleavers

Homeopathy

- Psorinum
- Sulfur
- Graphites

Juice Therapy

- Apple and carrot
- Beet, cucumber, and grape
- No citrus

<u>RASHES</u>

Nutritional Therapy
- Avoid citrus fruits
- Avoid berries
- Avoid peanuts
- Avoid shellfish
- Avoid dairy products

Vitamin/Mineral Therapy
- Vitamin A
- Vitamin C
- Vitamin E
- Flaxseed oil

Herbal Therapy
- Burdock root
- Gentian root
- Fresh aloe vera gel or juice

Juice Therapy
- Fresh vegetable juice
- Fresh fruit juice
- Wheatgrass juice

RAYNAUD'S DISEASE

Nutritional Therapy
- Raw seeds
- Hot vegetable soups
- Avoid coffee

Vitamin/Mineral Therapy
- Vitamin E (1,000 - 1,500 IU daily)
- Magnesium (200 mg three times daily)
- Folic acid (1g daily)
- Evening primrose oil (1,000 mg)

Herbal Therapy
- Ginkgo biloba
- Prickly ash
- Ginger

Homeopathy
- Arsen alb
- Secale

Juice Therapy
- Fresh fruit juices
- Fresh Vegetable juices

RESPIRATORY CONDITIONS

Nutritional Therapy
- A vegan diet
- Avoid alcohol
- Eat garlic
- Eat onion
- Drink plenty of water

Vitamin/Mineral Therapy
- Beta carotene
- Vitamin B6
- Vitamin C
- Vitamin E
- Calcium
- Chromium Picolinate
- Selenium
- Omega-3 fatty acids
- Flaxseed oil

Herbal Therapy
- Echinacea
- Goldenseal
- Mullein

Other
- 20 minutes of aerobic exercise
- Explore thoughts, attitudes, & beliefs, as well as improperly expressed emotions.
- Periodic fasting
- Hot water and lemon juice

RINGWORM

Nutritional Therapy
- A low sugar diet
- Cook with garlic

Vitamin/Mineral Therapy
- Vitamin A
- Vitamin B Complex
- Vitamin C with bioflavonoids
- Citrus seed extract
- Bee pollen

Herbal Therapy
- Myrrh powder
- Goldenseal powder

Homeopathy
- Sepia
- Arsen alb
- Graphites

Juice Therapy
- Strawberry and date juice (use fresh dates)

<u>SEXUALLY TRANSMITTED DISEASE</u>

Herbal Therapy
- Sarsaparilla
- Yellow Dock

Homeopathy
- Rhus tox
- Sepia
- Natrum mur
- Hepar sulph
- Arsen alb
- Caladium

Juice Therapy
- Carrot, beet, celery juice
- Avoid citrus and pineapple

Topical Therapy
- Vitamin C paste
- Tea tree oil diluted with water

Aromatherapy
- Tea tree
- Bergamot
- Eucalyptus
- Lavender
- Chamomile

SCIATICA

Nutritional Therapy

- Dark green leafy vegetables
- Yellow vegetables
- Whole grains
- Raw seeds and nuts

Vitamin/Mineral Therapy

- Magnesium
- Vitamin B1 (thiamin)
- Vitamin B Complex
- Vitamin E
- Manganese sulfate

Herbal Therapy

- Willow bark
- St. John's Wort
- Black Cohosh
- Fenugreek
- Parsley

Homeopathy

- Colocynth
- Viscum album
- Lachesis
- Rhus tox
- Lycopodium
- Ruta grav

SHINGLES (HERPES ZOSTER)

Nutritional Therapy
- Whole foods diet
- Avoid excessive refined carbohydrates

Vitamin/Mineral Therapy
- Vitamin B12 injections
- L-Lysine (4-5 g for two days then 500 mg two times daily for several weeks only)
- Vitamin C (6,000 mg divided into 1,000 mg doses)

Herbal Therapy
- Oat straw
- St. John's Wort
- Skullcap

Homeopathy
- Arsen alb
- Rhus tox
- Sepia
- Natrum mur
- Hepar sulph
- Caladium

Juice Therapy
- Carrot, celery, parsley
- Spinach, beet

SLEEP DISORDERS

Nutritional Therapy
- Reduce alcohol consumption
- Avoid all forms of caffeine
- Eat more protein and less carbs

Vitamin/Mineral Therapy
- Vitamin B12

Herbal Therapy
- Melatonin
- Chamomile
- Skullcap
- Valerian
- Hops
- Kava-kava

Juice Therapy
- Carrot, spinach, lettuce, celery juice

Other
- Do not spend a lot of time in bed trying to fall asleep
- Do not read, watch television, or use electronics in bed

SORE THROAT

Nutritional Therapy
- Increase fluid intake
- Drink hot herbal teas
- Drink broths
- Drink hot lemon water with honey
- Avoid refined sugar

Vitamin/Mineral Therapy
- Vitamin C with bioflavonoids
- Vitamin A (triple doses for first few days)
- Zinc
- Vitamin C

Herbal Therapy
- Gargle with sage or licorice
- Gargle with essential tea tree oil
- Ginger
- Echinacea
- Goldenseal

Homeopathy
- Lachesis
- Ignatia
- Arnica
- Aconite

Juice Therapy
- Juice of red potato

SPORTS INJURIES

Nutritional Therapy
- Whole foods diet (75% until healed)
- Green leafy vegetables
- Drink plenty of water

Vitamin/Mineral Therapy
- Vitamin E
- Vitamin C
- Magnesium
- For bone fracture - selenium, coenzyme Q10, glutathione, chlorella, spirulina, green tea, ginseng, germanium

Herbal Therapy
- Valerian root
- Passionflower
- White willow bark
- Turmeric
- Boswellia

Homeopathy
- Arnica

Juice Therapy
- Raw fresh vegetable juice

SPRAINS

Nutritional Therapy
- Whole foods diet with plenty of fresh fruits
- Vegetables
- Nuts
- Seeds
- Whole grains

Vitamin/Mineral Therapy
- Bromelain
- Vitamin C

Herbal Therapy
- Horsetail
- Nettle
- Willow bark

Homeopathy
- Ruta grav

Juice Therapy
- Raw fresh vegetable juice
- Beet, radish, garlic, comfrey tea

STIES

Nutritional Therapy
- Whole foods diet
- Cook with garlic
- Avoid refined sugars

Vitamin/Mineral Therapy
- Vitamin A (100,000 IU daily for first 2 days then reduce to 50,000 IU daily for next few days, then 25,000 IU daily for one week?
- Vitamin C
- Beta carotene (50,000 IU daily for first few days)

Herbal Therapy
- Eye wash made with filtered eyebright and goldenseal
- Drink red raspberry tea

Homeopathy
- Pulsatilla
- Hepar sulph
- Sulfur
- Graphites

<u>STRESS</u>

Nutritional Therapy

- Avoid caffeine
- Avoid food additives
- Eat a diet high in complex carbohydrates

Vitamin/Mineral Therapy

- Vitamin B6
- Vitamin A
- Vitamin C
- Vitamin E

Herbal Therapy

- Passionflower
- Valerian Root
- American Ginseng

Aromatherapy

- Bergamot
- Frankincense
- Juniper
- Lavender
- Lemon
- Neroli
- Sandalwood

Other

- Walking
- Stretching
- Plenty of sleep
- Laughter

STROKE

Nutritional Therapy

- Eat plenty of garlic
- Eat plenty of onions
- Avoid deep fried foods
- Eat raw nuts
- Eat raw seeds
- Avoid alcohol and alcohol binges (more than four drinks in a short period of time)

Vitamin/Mineral Therapy

- Vitamin E (triple the dosage for first few days then decrease)
- Omega-3 fatty acids
- Vitamin B6
- Magnesium
- Vitamin C

Herbal Therapy

- Elderberry
- Rosemary
- Damiana
- Siberian ginseng
- Lavender

SUNBURN

Vitamin/Mineral Therapy
- Vitamin E
- Vitamin A
- Vitamin C
- Potassium (100 mg daily for one to two weeks)

Herbal Therapy
- Aloe vera gel
- St. John's Wort
- Calendula flowers

Homeopathy
- Natrum mur
- Urtica urens
- Rhus tox

Juice Therapy
- Carrot juice

Other Therapy
- Bathe with apple cider vinegar

SWELLING

Nutritional Therapy
- Whole foods diet
- Decrease salt
- Limit commercial sodas
- Avoid refined sugars

Vitamin/Mineral Therapy
- Bromelain (on an empty stomach)
- Vitamin C with bioflavonoids
- Vitamin B Complex

Herbal Therapy
- Ginger root

Homeopathy
- Belladonna
- Aconite
- Ferrum phos
- Sulfur

Juice Therapy
- Fresh pineapple juice
- Carrot, celery, cucumber

<u>TENDINITIS</u>

Nutritional Therapy
- Avoid white potatoes
- Avoid tomatoes
- Avoid eggplant
- Avoid all peppers except black

Vitamin/Mineral Therapy
- Vitamin B6
- Vitamin B Complex
- Vitamin C with bioflavonoids
- Copper orally (2-4 mg daily) and/or wear a copper bracelet
- Manganese
- Bromelain
- Selenium

Herbal Therapy
- Willow bark
- Cramp bark

Homeopathy
- Aconite
- Thuja
- Ruta grav
- Belladonna
- Apis mel

TONSILLITIS

Nutritional Therapy
- Lots of fluids
- Warm broths
- Eat honey and lemon juice

Vitamin/Mineral Therapy
- Vitamin A (100,000 IU first 3 days, then 25,000 for the next week)
- Zinc
- Vitamin B Complex
- Vitamin C
- Garlic capsules

Herbal Therapy
- Cleavers
- Echinacea
- Elderflower
- Yarrow

Homeopathy
- Belladonna
- Merc sol
- Phytolacca
- Lachesis
- Aconite

Juice Therapy
- Carrot, beet and tomato
- Carrot, pineapple

TUBERCULOSIS

Nutritional Therapy
- Whole foods
- Plenty of raw foods
- Plenty of fluids
- Eat pears daily

Vitamin/Mineral Therapy
- Vitamin A (300,000 IU for first three days, then 200,000 IU next two days then 50,000 IU for several weeks)
- Beta carotene (25,000 - 50,000 IU)
- Vitamin E (increase up to 1,000 IU daily unless peri/menopausal)
- Vitamin B Complex

Herbal Therapy
- Echinacea
- Mullein
- Garlic capsules (three times a day)

Juice Therapy
- Pear juice
- Raw potato juice (allow starch to settle and use the juice)
- Carrot juice and olive or almond oil

Topical Therapy
- Eucalyptus oil packs
- Grape packs

URINARY PROBLEMS

Nutritional Therapy
- Pure cranberry juice
- Avoid coffee
- Avoid artificial sweeteners
- Avoid carbonated beverages
- Avoid tomato-based foods

Vitamin/Mineral Therapy
- Vitamin C
- Baking soda (½ tsp mixed with water)
- Vitamin B1 (30-50 mg two to three times per day between meals for one week)

Herbal Therapy
- Nettle
- Horsetail
- Fennel
- Echinacea
- Juniper berries
- Skullcap

Homeopathy
- Aconite
- Cantharis

Juice Therapy
- Carrot, parsley, celery, cucumber
- Cranberry juice

VARICOSE VEINS

Nutritional Therapy
- Bowel cleansing program
- Drink lots of pure water
- Eat berries and cherries
- Eat organic citrus fruits
- Eat garlic, onions, and ginger
- Avoid cheese

Vitamin/Mineral Therapy
- Rutin (1 g per day for up to 1 year)
- Vitamin C (taken throughout the day)
- Vitamin B Complex
- Vitamin B6 (30 -100 mg daily for 3 -4 months)
- Vitamin E (400 IU)
- Vitamin D (500 mg daily for two months)

Herbal Therapy
- Hawthorn
- Ginkgo
- Prickly Ash

Homeopathy
- Calc fluor
- Hamamelis

Juice Therapy
- Carrot, celery, and parsley
- Carrot, spinach, and turnip

VERTIGO

Nutritional Therapy
- Avoid caffeine
- Avoid salt
- Avoid fried foods
- Avoid aspartame

Vitamin/Mineral Therapy
- Vitamin B Complex
- Vitamin C plus bioflavonoids
- Choline (500 mg two times daily)
- Vitamin E

Herbal Therapy
- Ginkgo (40 mg three times a day)
- Ginger (1 capsule three times a day)

Homeopathy
- Gelsemium
- Phosphorus
- Cocculus
- Aconite
- Sulfur
- Silicea
- Lycopodium
- Belladonna

VIRAL INFECTIONS

Nutritional Therapy
- Whole foods diet

Vitamin/Mineral Therapy
- Vitamin C (3,000 mg daily)
- Vitamin A
  Vitamin B Complex
- Pantothenic acid (1 -3 g two to three times daily)
- L-cysteine

Herbal Therapy
- Echinacea
- Goldenseal
- Myrrh
- Astragalus
- Garlic

Homeopathy
- Calendula
- Chamomilla
- Belladonna
- Sulfur

Juice Therapy
- Carrot, celery, beet, garlic

VISION DISORDERS

Nutritional Therapy
- Unrefined foods
- Avoid alcohol
- Eliminate sugar
- Eat dark leafy green vegetables
- Eat red, blue, and purple fruits

Vitamin/Mineral Therapy
- Xincer
- Selenium
- Taurine
- Vitamin C
- Vitamin E
- N-acetyl-cysteine
- Ginkgo biloba

Herbal Therapy
- Ginkgo biloba
- Grape Seed Extract
- Pine bark
- Siberian ginseng

Juice Therapy
- Fresh carrot juice
- Carrot juice with celery, parsley, spinach or cucumber

Other
- Use a raw-potato eye pack
- Cucumber wash

VOMITING

Nutritional Therapy
- Drink fluids
- Avoid solid foods
- Avoid dairy
- Eat light vegetable broth after vomiting has subsided
- Resume normal diet after 2 -3 days

Vitamin/Mineral Therapy
- Wait one day after vomiting has stopped to take supplements
- Folic Acid (400- 500 mcg two to three times daily)
- Vitamin A (10,000 IU)
- Vitamin B1 (50 mg)

Homeopathy
- Ipecac
- Phosphorus
- Arsen alb
- Nux vom

Juice Therapy
- Any vegetable juice with added ginger

<u>WARTS</u>

Nutritional Therapy
- Dark green vegetables
- Yellow vegetables
- Eat onions
- Eat garlic
- Eat brussel sprouts
- Eat cabbage

Vitamin/Mineral Therapy
- Vitamin A (100,000 IU for five days, then reduce to 25,000 IU for one month)
- Beta carotene (50,000 IU for several weeks)
- L-cysteine (500 mg two times daily for one month with an amino acid blend one time daily)
- Vitamin B Complex

Herbal Therapy
- Dandelion stem (apply the milky substance squeezed from stem to wart twice daily)

Homeopathy
- Thuja
- Causticum
- Calc carb
- Ruta grav
- Graphites

WHOOPING COUGH

Nutritional Therapy
- Drink plenty of fluids
- Drink 1 tablespoon apple cider vinegar with 1 tablespoon honey and fresh lemon juice with warm water.
- Avoid all dairy products

Vitamin/Mineral Therapy
- Zinc lozenges
- Vitamin C
- Vitamin A (200,000 IU first three days, 100,000 IU next three days, then 25,000 IU for several months)
- Beta carotene (50,000 IU daily for one month, then 25,000 IU daily)

Herbal Therapy
- Thyme
- Wild cherry bark
- Anise

Homeopathy
- Drosera
- Pertussinum
- Cuprum met
- Mag phos

Juice Therapy
- Orange, lemon
- Carrot, watercress

WORMS

Nutritional Therapy

- Whole foods diet
- Eat pumpkin seeds
- Eat papaya seeds
- Eat pineapple

Vitamin/Mineral Therapy

- Vitamin C
- Beta carotene

Herbal Therapy

- Aloe vera gel or juice (twice daily on an empty stomach)

Juice Therapy

- Pineapple juice

WOUNDS

Nutritional Therapy
- Eat green vegetables
- Eat yellow vegetables
- Eat raw seeds and nuts

Vitamin/Mineral Therapy
- Vitamin A (50,000 IU daily for several weeks)
- Zinc (30 - 60 mg)
- Vitamin B - Pantothenic acid (500 mg twice daily)
- Vitamin C
- Vitamin B Complex

Herbal Therapy
- Calendula ointment
- Echinacea ointment
- Goldenseal ointment
- Apply witch hazel

Homeopathy Therapy
- Calendula
- Hypericum
- Ledum

Juice Therapy
- Beet
- Carrot
- Celery

ALTERNATIVES TO ANTIBIOTICS

Herbal Therapy

- Garlic
- Echinacea
- Goldenseal
- Astragalus
- Panax ginseng
- Reishi mushroom
- Shiitake mushroom
- Slippery elm

Vitamin Therapy

- Selenium
- Vitamins A, B, C

Essential Oils Therapy

- Tea Tree oil
- Thyme
- Eucalyptus
- Geranium

Homeopathic Therapy

- Apis mellifica
- Arsenicum album
- Belladonna
- Rhus toxicodendron
- Hepar sulphuris

9 781985 877504